My Ramadan Gratitude Moments

Written and Illustrated by S. Samia Quddus

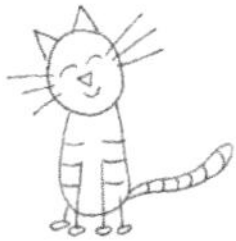

Dedicated to Simba for bringing so much joy

With special thanks to Dr. Sheikh Saalim Al-Azhari, Shaheen Bilgrami and Calley Dickinson (MBACP)

First published in Great Britain in 2022 by Deft Group Publishing Plc.
187a Hertford Road, London, United Kingdom, N9 7EP
www.deftgroupltd.co

A CIP catalogue record for this book is available from the British Library
ISBN Number 978-1-3999-1001-9
All papers used by Deft Group Ltd are natural, recyclable products
made from wood grown in well managed forests.
Designed by The Grid @designthegrid | Printed in Great Britain

Contents

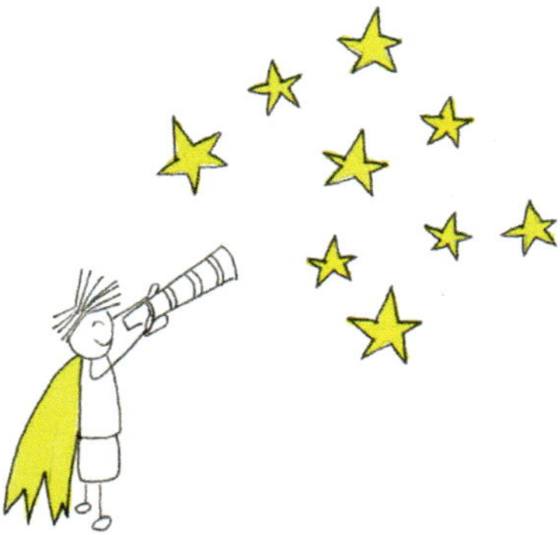

This book belongs to:

....

Date:

....

How To Use This Book

Salaams and welcome!

This book will help you:

- Learn how gratitude can make you happier and can improve your life!
- Find out about the effects of gratitude on your brain and body
- Complete 30 gratitude activities on the 30 days of Ramadan
- Find something to be grateful for in different situations
- Understand when to say *Alhamdulillah*
- Get closer to Allah during Ramadan
- Connect with your loved ones in new and different ways
- Learn to find something to be grateful for, even on the not-so-good days!

In short, this book will help you to become happier by learning to live a life filled with positivity and gratitude. Each activity will help to build your 'gratitude muscle'. Find a Gratitude Buddy to help if you get stuck!

What is GRATITUDE?

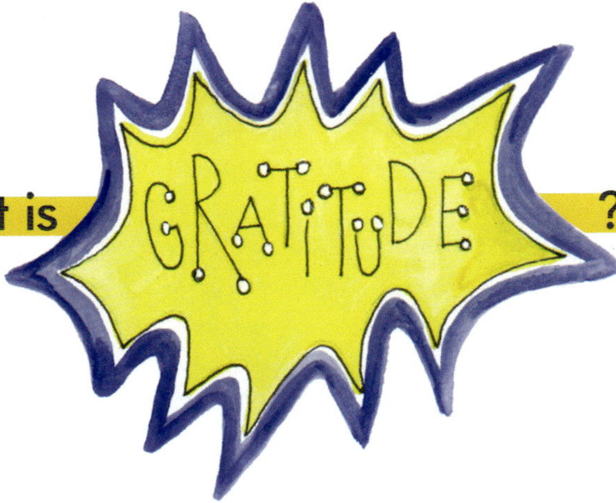

Gratitude is a feeling and a way of thinking. We show gratitude by giving thanks. Saying "thank you" is just one way of expressing gratitude. There are many different ways we can speak about gratitude. Here are just a few ways...

I am grateful for...

I am thankful for...

I am appreciative for...

How to Show Gratitude?

You can show gratitude in your actions, by giving gifts, compliments, hugs, and smiles, and by helping others. You can feel grateful for important people in your life, your possessions and things which make you happy. Did you know that you can also search for the good, even when things feel difficult?

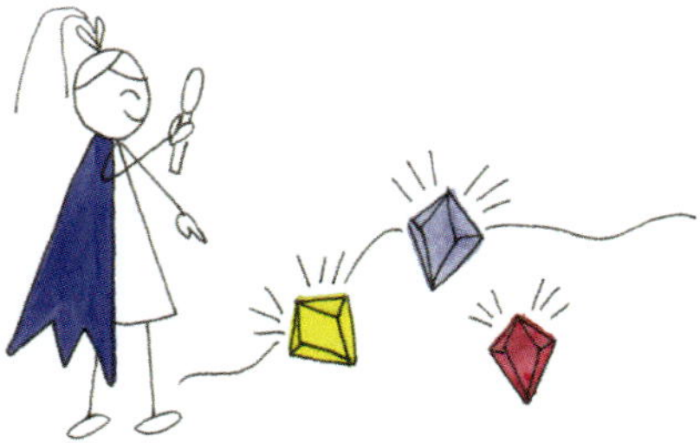

For example, when you've had a fight with someone special, or when you didn't get what you wanted for Eid. Here, the good isn't clear to see, but if you look hard enough, you *will* find something to be grateful for. So, you could think, at least you have someone special to fight with, who you can also have fun with, and, at least you have people to give you Eid gifts.

The more you practice gratitude, the stronger your gratitude muscle becomes, which makes it easier to feel grateful. When you feel grateful, you think in a way that is positive and hopeful. This creates an ***"attitude of gratitude"***.

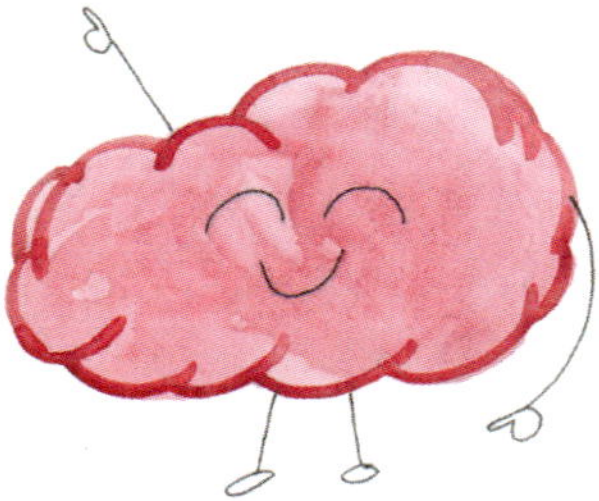

Gratitude and the Brain

Let me tell you a secret, gratitude is a superpower! When we feel grateful, we can change the way other people feel and how we feel.

And when we feel grateful, something amazing happens to our brain... It releases two happy chemicals called Dopamine and Serotonin.

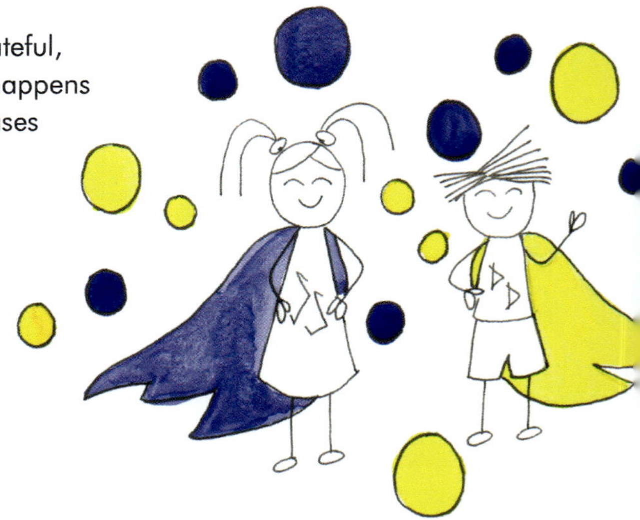

Let's imagine them as superheroes! ***Meet Dynamic Dopamine and Super Serotonin.***

Dynamic Dopamine and Super Serotonin are released from different parts of the brain to work together. **This makes us feel happy and positive.** The more we focus on being grateful for things, the better our brain becomes at discovering other things to be grateful for.

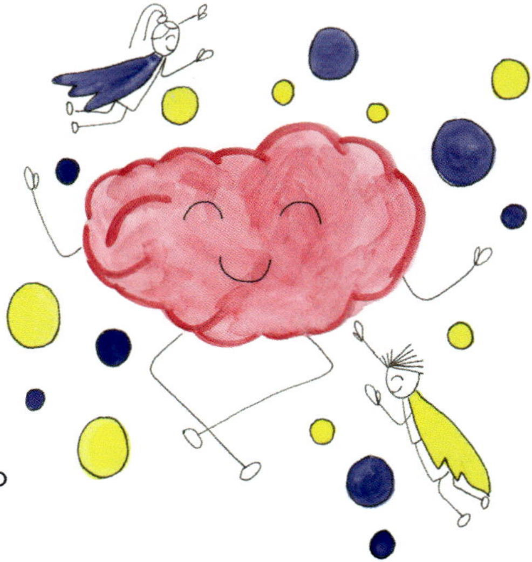

This helps us to keep feeling happy. When we feel happy, we feel grateful for the things that are making us happy. The great thing is that everyone can show and feel gratitude.

Remember, the more you feel grateful, the more Dynamic Dopamine and Super Serotonin are released which results in a happier you! So, all you need to do to be happier is to practice feeling grateful. **You can do it!**

Gratitude as a Muslim

Gratitude is so important for Muslims that it even has its own special word in Arabic. Do you know what the word is? Fill in the blank letters if you know. The answer is at the bottom of the page if you don't know!

sh _ _ r

Allah's name Is Ash-Shakur

Did you know that one of Allah's special names is *Ash-Shakur,* The Grateful, The Appreciative? When we are grateful to Allah for all that we have, and we show appreciation for everything He has created (including the people we really care about like our parents, siblings and relatives), He rewards us. ***That's how important being thankful and appreciative is to Allah.***

The answer is 'shukr'

appreciate

grateful

Other Words for Gratitude

thankful

shukr (Arabic)

Can you think of any more?

When we Say *Alhamdulillah*

Most of the time, we say, *'Alhamdulillah'* when we want to praise Allah and thank Him for everything in our life. We often say *Alhamdulillah* for someone getting well after being sick. We also say *Alhamdulillah* during difficult times, like when things don't go the way we want it to or when we hear sad news.

There are so many times to praise Allah, some that you might not have thought about before. We can call these, *Alhamdulillah* moments. Every day in the month of Ramadan, we'll help you to think about some special *Alhamdulillah* moments.

Remember the idea of gratitude being a bit like a superpower? When we say *Alhamdulillah*, it helps us to feel close to Allah and to connect with Him. This makes us feel happy. Here's another super special fact. Did you know that Allah will give us more when we are grateful?

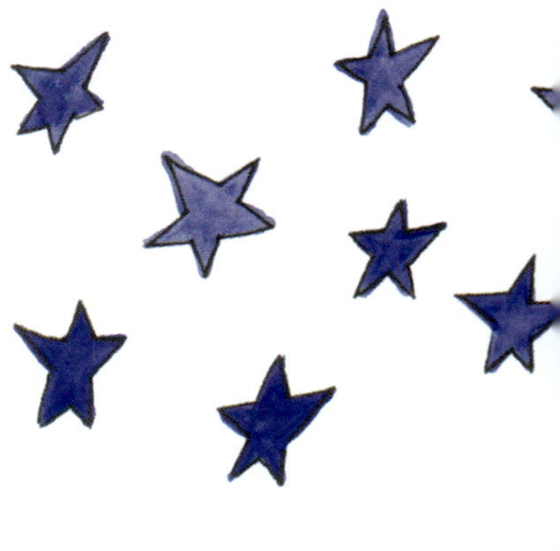

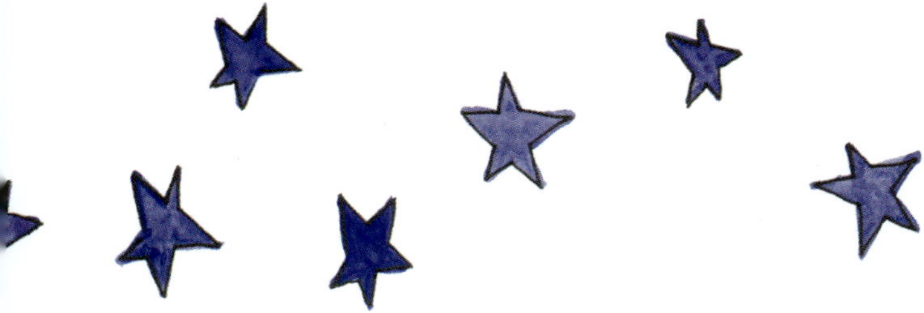

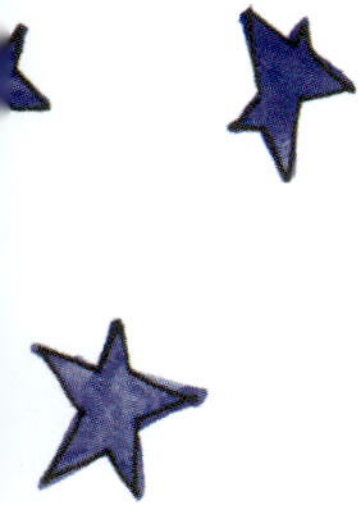

Allah says,

"If you are grateful, I will give you more."

(Surah Al-Ibrahim, Verse 7).

That's His promise to us. How wonderful is that? This shows us the importance of living with gratitude as Muslims. The more we can see things through grateful eyes, the more we will recognise all the good in our life, even during the times that appear not so good. Allah mentions the importance of being grateful many times in the Qur'an. He reminds us that we can use our blessings to help others and that He will reward us for our generosity.

Gratitude and Our Community

Gratitude also helps us build strong relationships with everyone around us, especially the people we love. This is great because, as Muslims, living harmoniously with our families and everyone in our communities is very important.

Can you see how much of a superpower gratitude, or *shukr* as it is called in Arabic, really is?

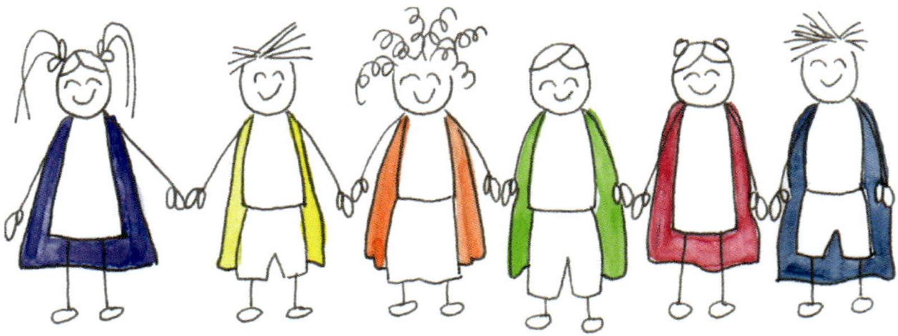

Gratitude and Ramadan

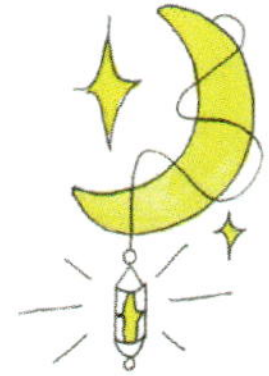

Ramadan is the perfect time to show *shukr* (gratitude). Allah created us to worship Him, remember Him and to express *shukr* to Him. Identifying our blessings, appreciating how fortunate we are and being thankful for all our situations are some of the ways we show shukr.

Ramadan is also a time to remember all the good things we have, to show extra kindness and help to make things better for others by supporting them in different ways. Remember the importance of caring for communities? These are the things that Allah loves and by doing these things, we can grow closer to Allah too.

My Ramadan Gratitude Moments will help you to think about positive *Alhamdulillah* moments that you can be grateful for everyday during Ramadan. We'll also give you some activity ideas you can do to explore your gratitude. That's thirty days of Ramadan gratitude moments! And it doesn't stop there – when the month of Ramadan ends, you will have learned to find *Alhamdulillah* moments in all sorts of places and situations, both expected and unexpected.

Your Mission...

To find and to feel positive about things in your life and to show appreciation to people and Allah. so that being grateful becomes a habit you can continue beyond Ramadan.

Remember that gratitude releases Dynamic Dopamine and Super Serotonin, so, they will be around, helping to keep you going along the way! Are you ready?

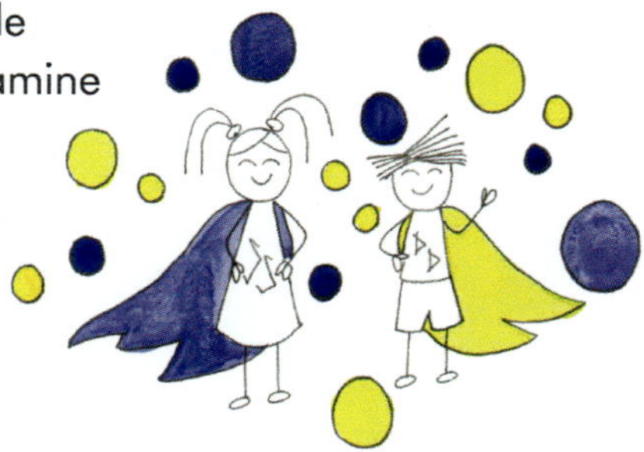

Bismillah. let's go!

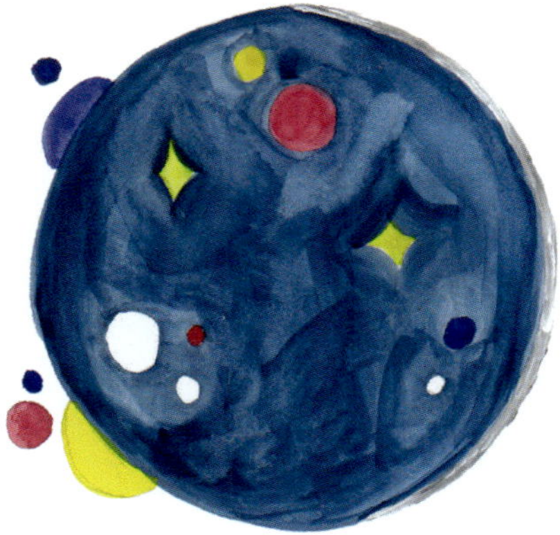

Day 1

It's the first day of Ramadan! What a wonderful blessing that we can take part in this holy month, *Alhamdulillah*.

Thank Allah for blessing you with Ramadan with all your heart. Write down what you are most looking forward to in this special month.

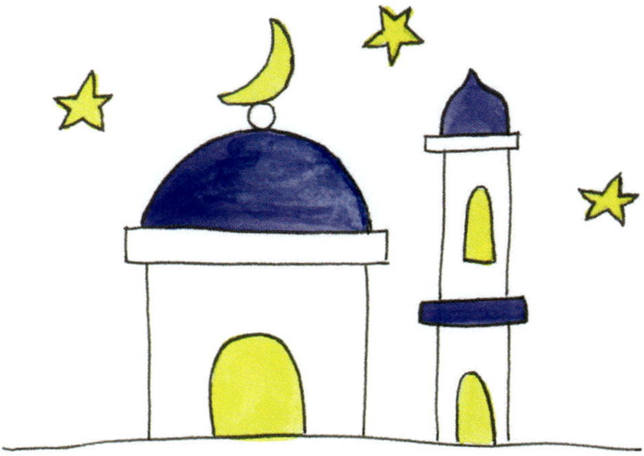

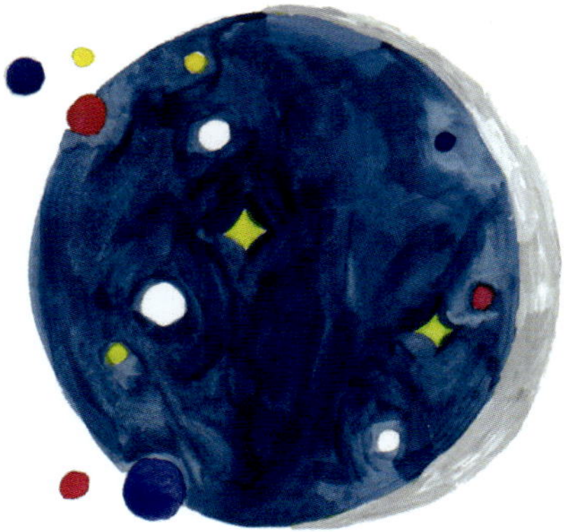

Day 2

Ramadan is a time to try our best to show Allah that we can be better Muslims, *Alhamdulillah*.

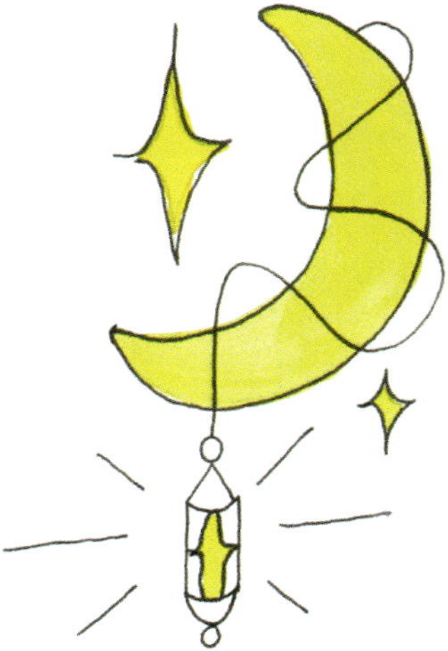

What do you like most about being a Muslim? Think about some of the traditions and celebrations that you enjoy. What makes them special for you? Remember to thank Allah!

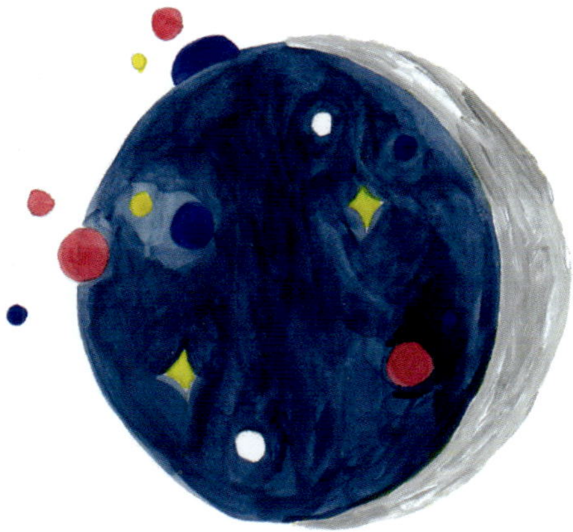

Day 3

Ramadan is a time when Allah gives us extra rewards for all our efforts, even if they are super small, *Alhamdulillah*.

Find a pea. Did you know that all good deeds are rewarded, even if they are the size of a pea?

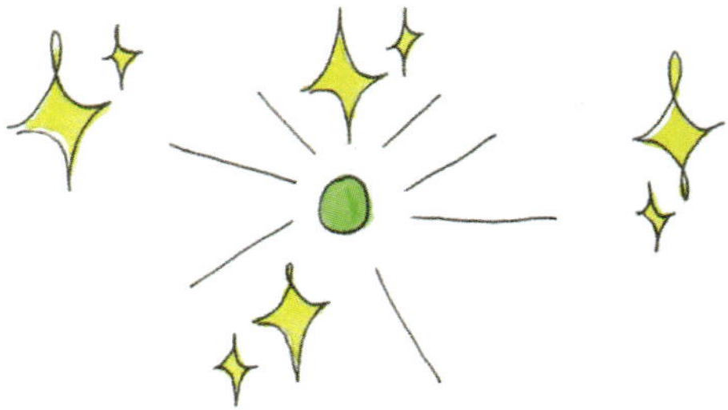

Collect a penny a day in a clear glass jar for **sadaqah** (charity). A penny might not seem like much, but it makes a big difference and carries a big reward when given to someone in need. When you collect a penny, every day for many days, it can add up to a lot of money and can help in important ways.

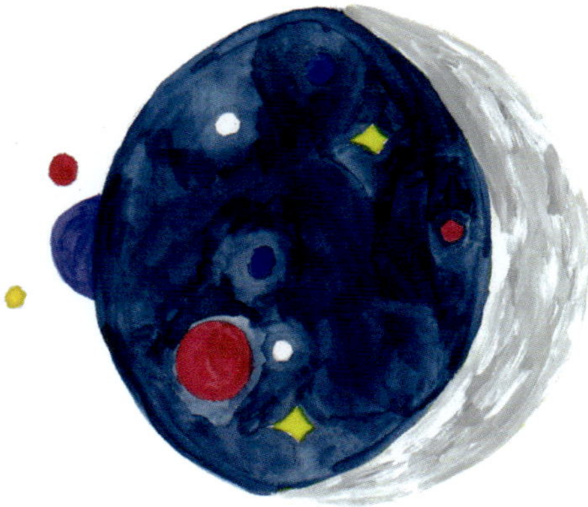

Day 4

Ramadan is a time to try and be extra close to Allah. Remember, He knows when we have made an effort to get closer to Him, *Alhamdulillah*.

Think about something you do that helps you to feel close to Allah.

Is it praying?
Is it reading the Qur'an?
Is it making a special **dua**?
Is it learning about Islam?
Is it saying a special word like **Alhamdulillah**?
Is it when you close your eyes and remember Allah?
Is it something else?

Finish this sentence: Thank you Allah for helping me feel close to you when I...

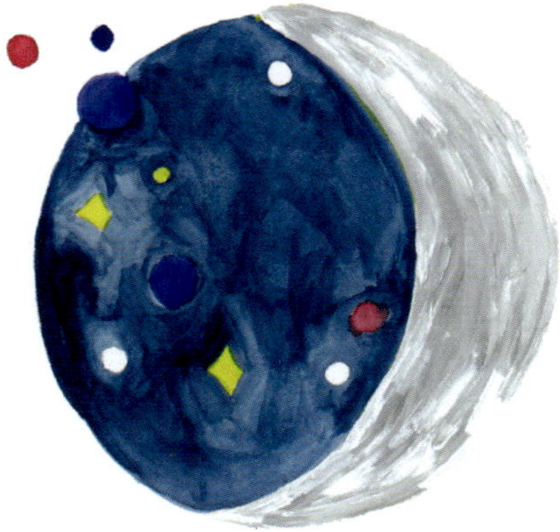

Day 5

Ramadan is a time to learn more about how to become a better Muslim. We have so many different things like books, toys, activities and people that we can learn from, *Alhamdulillah*.

Find your most favourite thing that helps you learn about Islam. What makes it so helpful?

If you could write a message to its maker, what would you say?

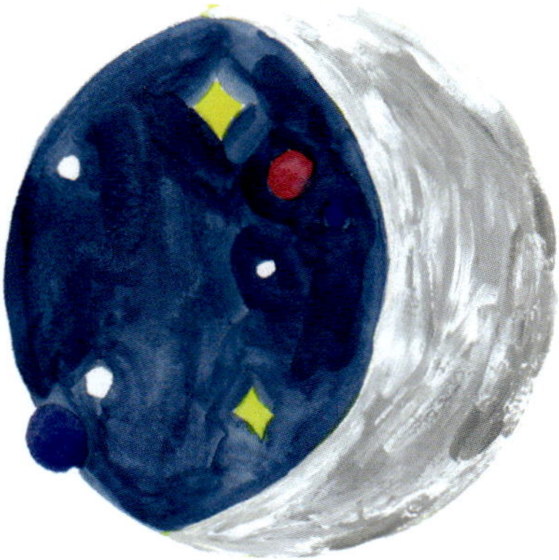

Day 6

Ramadan is a time when we can be extra helpful. Every helpful act is rewarded, *Alhamdulillah*.

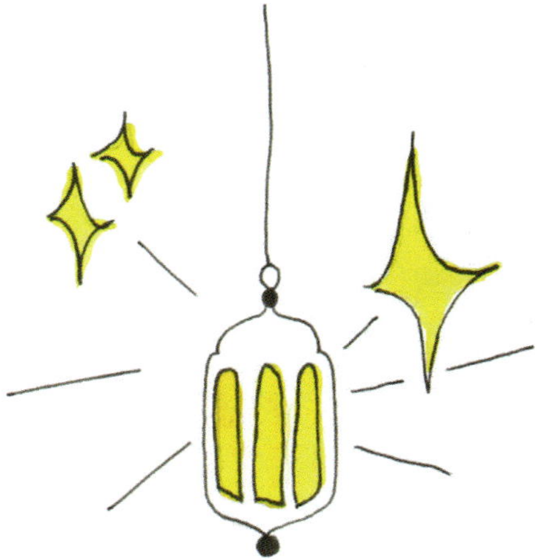

Think about the different ways you and the people in your family are helping others during Ramadan.

Can you imagine how this **feels** for others?

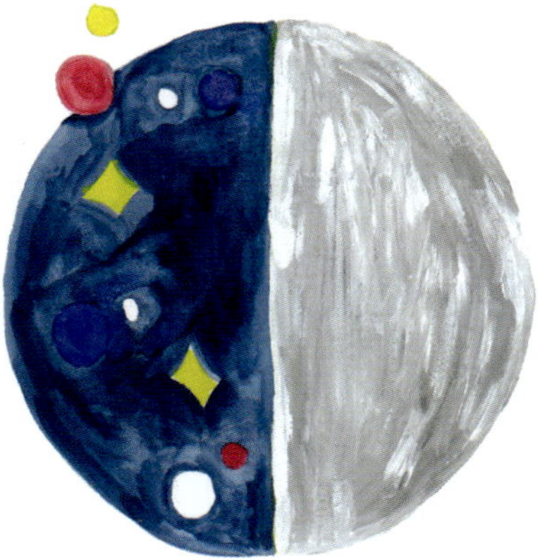

Day 7

Ramadan is a good time to think about our own positive qualities and how we can use them to help or inspire others, *Alhamdulillah!*

What qualities do you have that you are proud of? They could be kindness, honesty, humour, or something else.

Write a little thank you note to Allah explaining how these qualities He has given you have helped others around you.

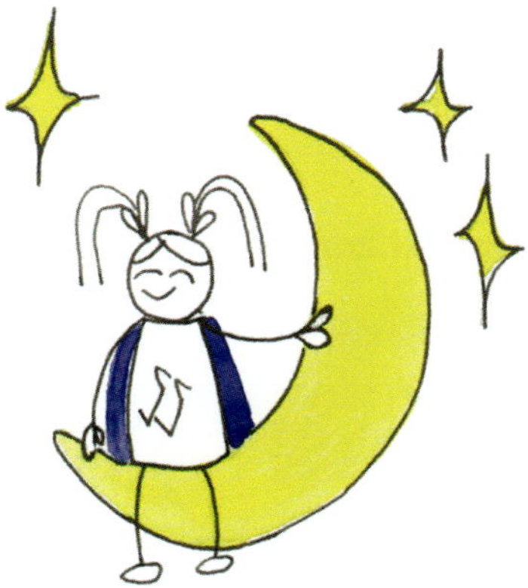

Thank Allah for giving you these amazing qualities.

Day 8

Ramadan is a time to remember and reflect on Allah's qualities. We can do this by finding out the meanings of His special names. Doing this will give us a deeper understanding of the awesomeness of Allah, and will make us feel happy, *Alhamdulillah*.

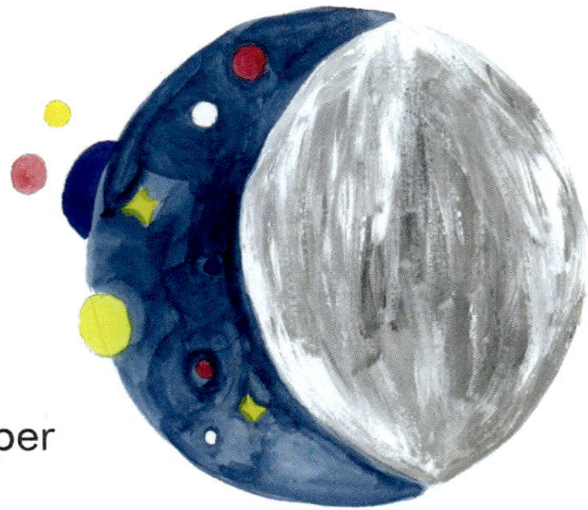

COOL FACT: Learning about Allah's qualities through His names can help us think about qualities we would like for ourselves.

Choose one of Allah's names, with an adult's help. Select a name that has a quality that you want to have. For example, to become kinder, choose **Ar Ra'oof**, meaning, 'The Most Kind'. Use this name in your dua to ask Allah to make you kinder. You can also practice being kind to others.

Some other names you might want to learn are Al Wadood, meaning 'The Most Loving', **Al Barr**, meaning 'The Source of Goodness', **Al Saboor**, meaning 'The Patient' and **Al Qawiyy**, meaning 'The Supremely Strong'.

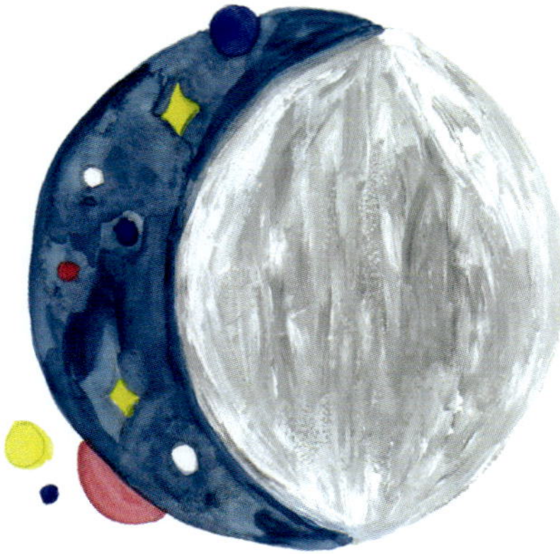

Day 9

Ramadan is a time to be generous! There are many different ways we can express generosity and the best thing is, Allah rewards every act of generosity (even if it's pea-sized), *Alhamdulillah*.

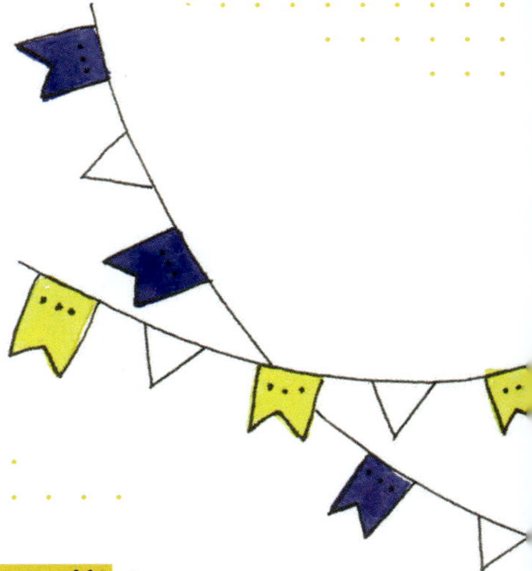

If you could create a unique gift for someone special, what would it be? How might the gift make your special someone **feel**?

Maybe it could be something they really want, or something that will make them happy, or maybe it's something they really need.

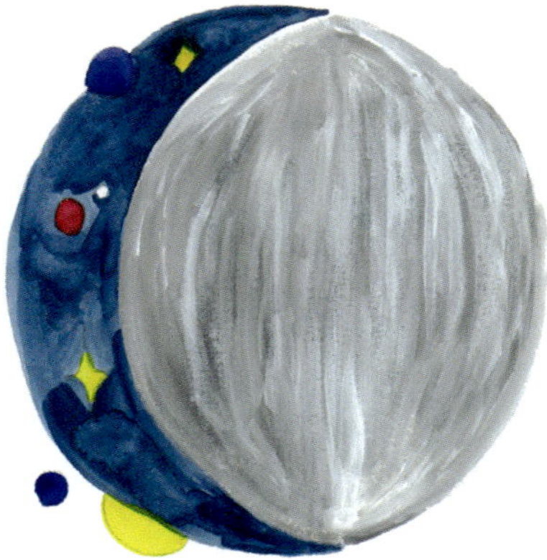

Day 10

You've been practicing gratitude for 10 days! That means Dynamic Dopamine and Super Serotonin have been releasing happy chemicals in your brain for 10 whole days, *Alhamdulillah!*

What have been your top three Ramadan **Alhamdulillah moments** so far? What has made them special?

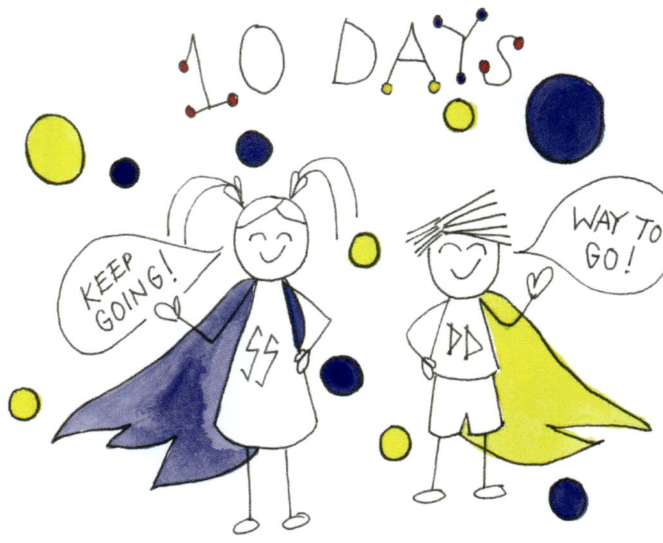

Day 11

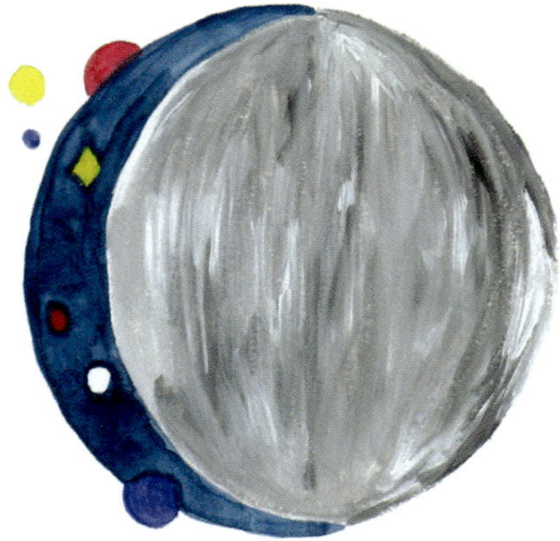

Ramadan is an amazing time to speak to Allah through your *duas*. Remember that you can feel as comfortable talking to Allah as someone close to you. Just as we can't see Dynamic Dopamine and Super Serotonin, but we know they are there, we know that Allah is always there, *Alhamdulillah*.

COOL FACT: Making *dua* is powerful. It's like an invisible superpower, because Allah listens and responds to all our *duas* in different ways.

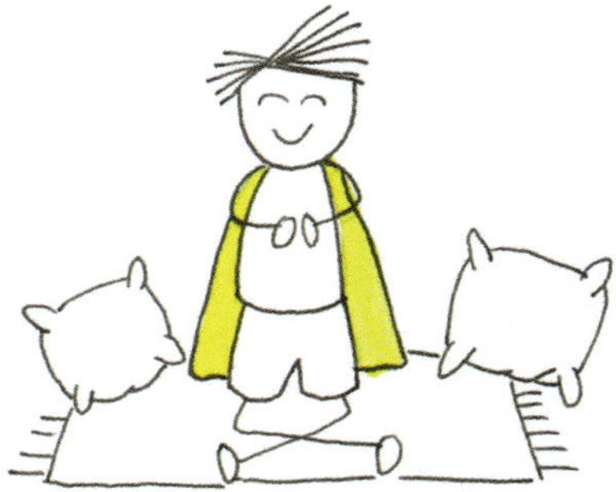

Do you have a favourite place in your home? Is it a place that is comfy and cosy? Is it a place where you can make **dua**? Close your eyes and imagine Allah is there.

What would you like to say to Allah? It can be anything. Maybe you can thank Him for giving you this favourite spot.

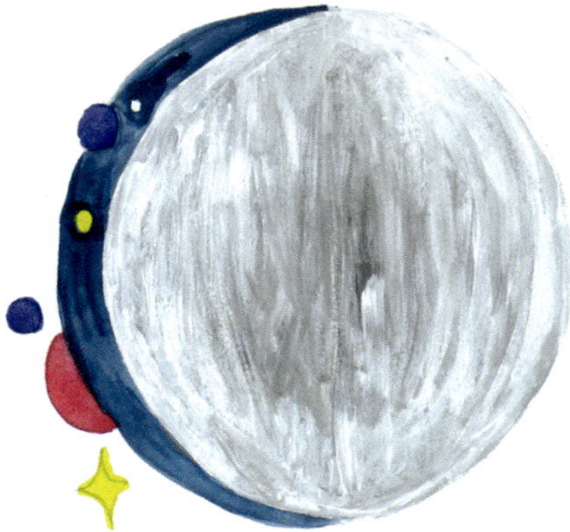

Day 12

Ramadan is a time to appreciate the things we own. This helps us to remember that Allah has given us different possessions and that we have a responsibility to look after them, *Alhamdulillah*.

Imagine if you had to leave your home and you could take one special thing that you really cared about, with you.

It could be a pet, a plant, a photograph, a special blanket or something else.

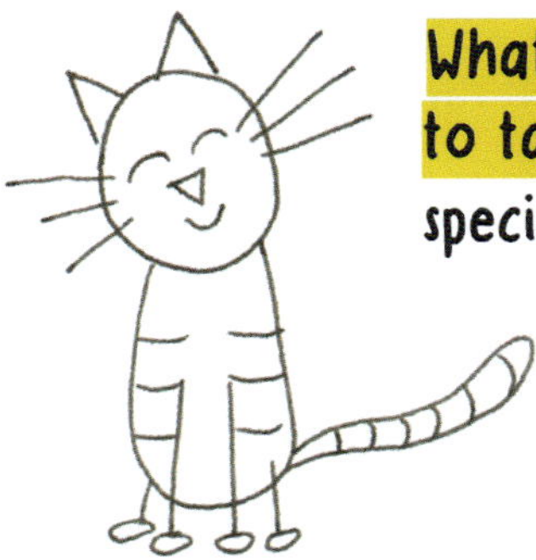

What would you choose to take? Why is this thing special to you?

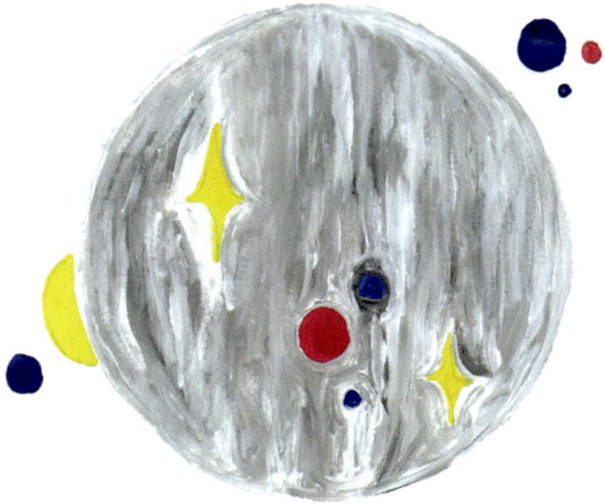

Day 13

Ramadan is a time to appreciate all the comforts that we already have. There are many children in the world who, despite having very little, say *Alhamdulillah* and thank Allah for all they have, even when they have fewer things than we do.

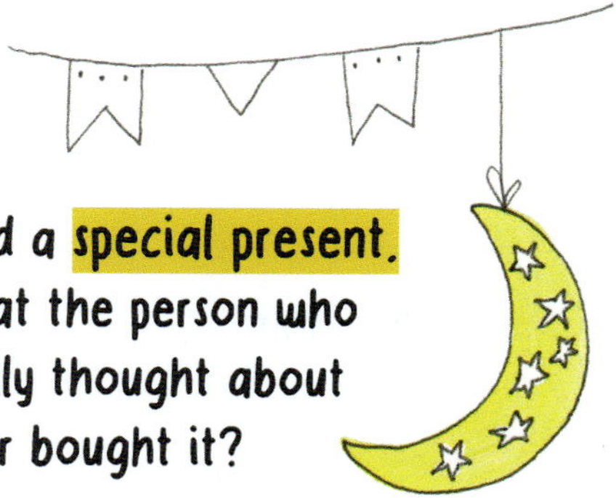

Have you ever received a special present that has shown you that the person who gave it to you has really thought about you when they made or bought it?

Ask a grown up to find a mosque or charity that is accepting Ramadan gifts for children whose families can't afford gifts. Now find a shoebox and fill it with presents for one of these children. Think carefully about the suitability of what you give and select things that you would love to receive yourself.

How would you like your shoebox gift to make someone **feel**?

Day 14

Ramadan is a time to appreciate things around us that we don't always notice. For example, things in nature, such as the different phases of the moon, or maybe the different shapes and colours of leaves or flowers.

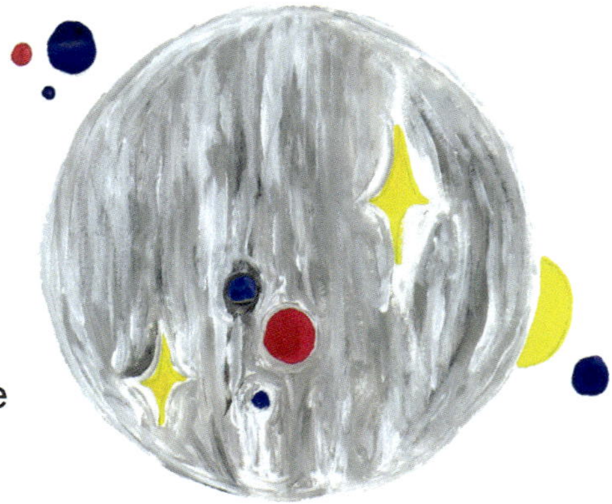

COOL FACT: Being in nature, surrounded by trees, grass and living things, is good for us. Super Serotonin is released when we are in nature. This helps us to feel happy and calm, *Alhamdulillah*.

Find a beautiful plant in your garden or in a park. Look at it closely and think about how Allah made this so perfectly, even if there are parts that don't seem perfect.

How do you think Allah might want you to feel when you look at it?

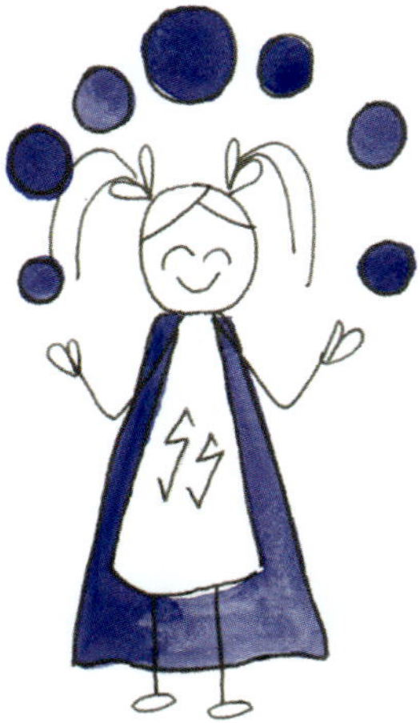

Allah made everything in nature to remind us of Him and for us to **feel** closer to Him. Whenever you see something impressive in nature that makes you feel **WOW** inside, you can say **"SubhanAllah"**.

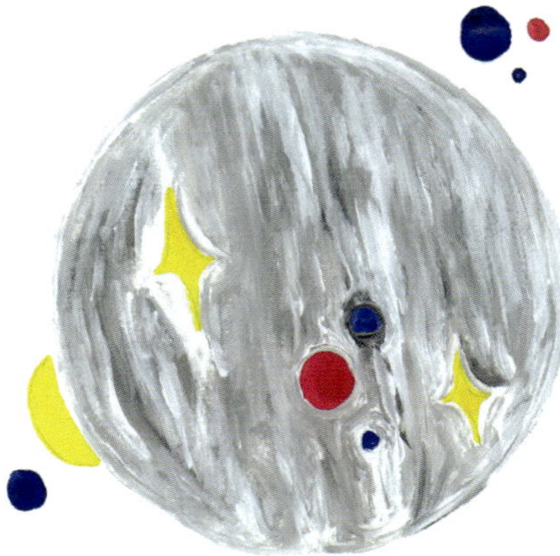

Day 15

Ramadan is a time to be thankful for all our food and drink, *Alhamdulillah*.

HERE'S A SUPER *ALHAMDULILLAH* FACT:
You receive the same reward when you feed a fasting person that you receive when you fast! How cool is that?

Choose someone special who you would like to feed (real or pretend).

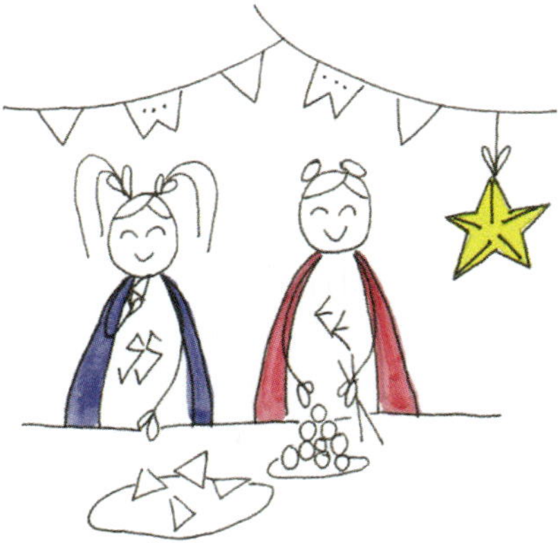

What would you prepare for them?
What would be special about your meal?
How do you hope making this meal will make them feel?

COOL FACT: What you eat affects your mood, so it's important to eat nutritious food that keeps you healthy and makes you feel good. This is because your tummy can produce even more Super Serotonin than your brain, so eating well will help you feel happy!

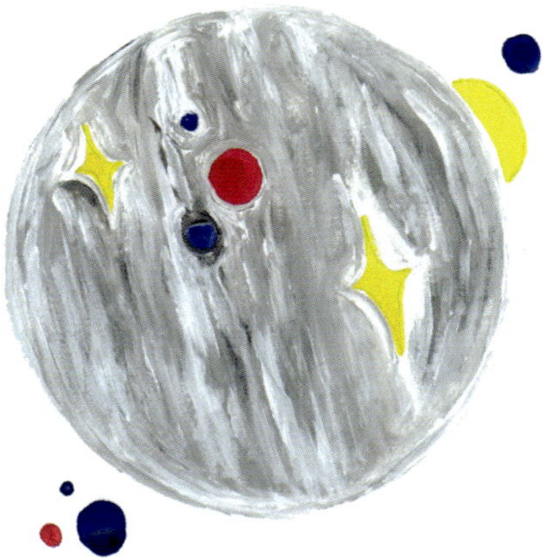

Day 16

Ramadan is a time to get closer to our families. Special moments spent praying, fasting and eating together will increase closeness, connection and love, *Alhamdulillah*.

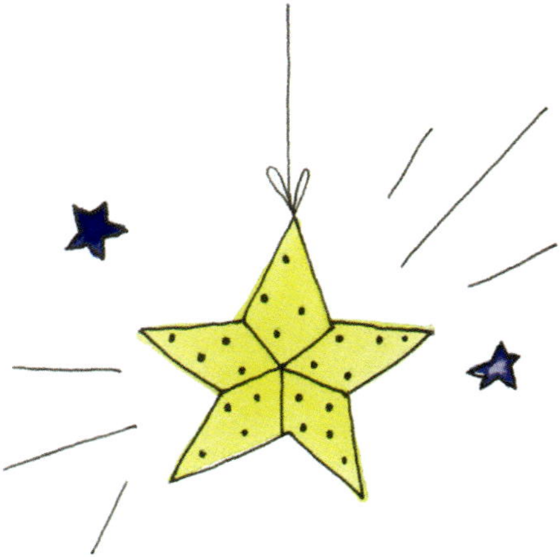

During Ramadan, is there a particular time of the day when your family comes together? What makes this time special for you?

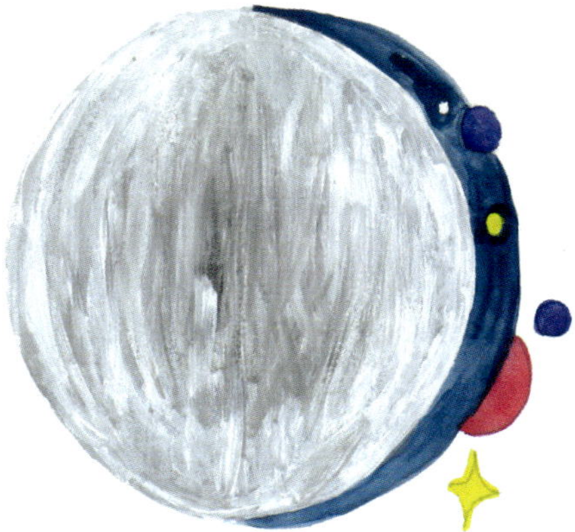

Day 17

Ramadan is a time when we can increase our prayers. Our prayers help us feel close to Allah during this blessed month, *Alhamdulillah*.

During Ramadan, lay out all the prayer mats for your family when it's time for prayer.

This is a small act which has a big reward, because you are helping your family prepare to connect with Allah through their prayers. How special is that?

Day 18

Ramadan is a time to remember and make *dua* for all the people we love no matter where they are. They might live with us, or near to us, or they might live far away. *Alhamdulillah*.

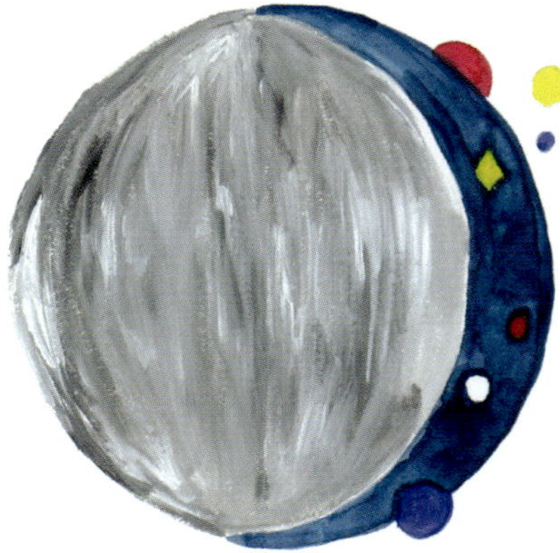

HERE'S A SUPER *ALHAMDULILLAH* FACT:
Every time you make *dua* for someone, Angels wish that same thing for you too. How special is that!?

Write a short dua for someone special who doesn't live with you. It could be for your grandmother, a cousin, a friend, or anyone you love.

Think about what the person you are making **dua** for needs, or likes and why.

Day 19

Ramadan is a time to be more friendly. You can start by smiling more. Smiling and being friendly will be rewarded both by Allah and by the people you smile at, *Alhamdulillah!*

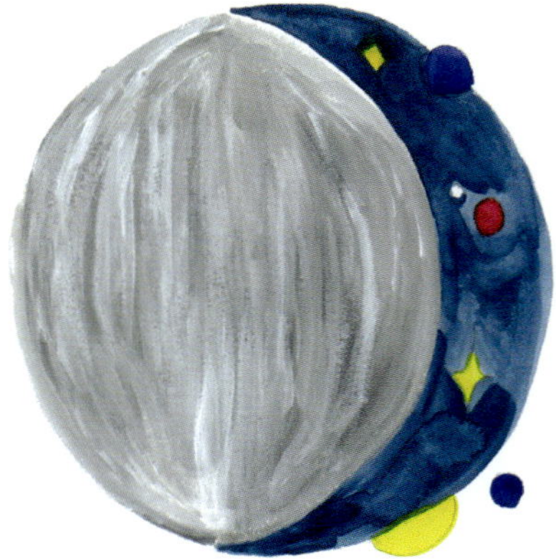

COOL FACT: When you smile, your brain also releases another happy chemical called Endorphin. We call it 'Epic Endorphin'. So, smiling releases Super Serotonin, Dynamic Dopamine and Epic Endorphin. They work together to help you feel happy, *Alhamdulillah!*

Make someone special smile every remaining day of Ramadan. You can even say a special **dua** for them **and** for others when you see them smile! Say, "**Adhakal Lahu Sinnaka.**" which means, 'May Allah always keep you smiling.' Isn't that beautiful?

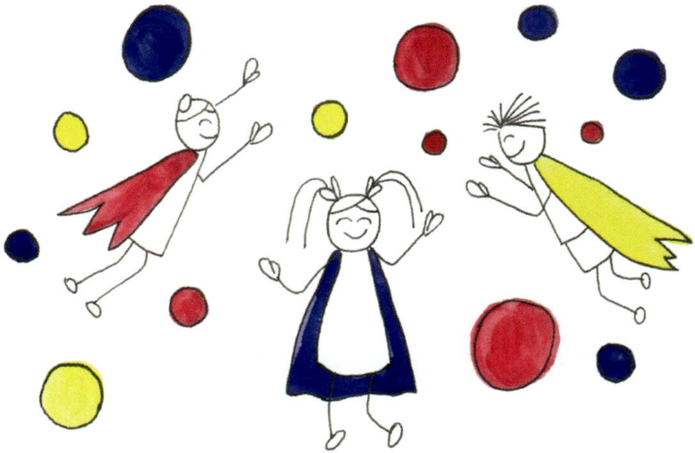

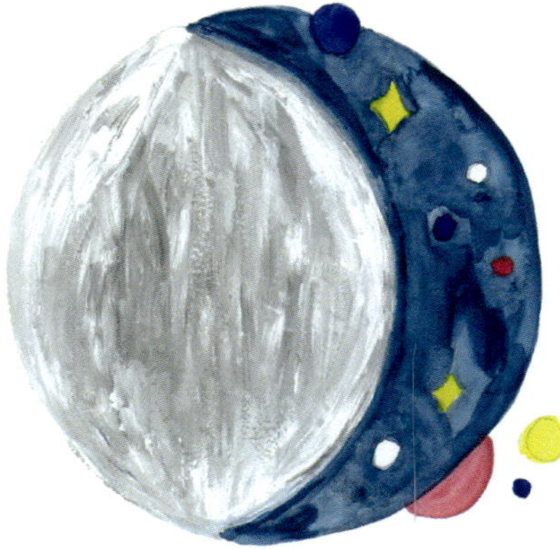

Day 20

Yay! You've been practicing gratitude for 20 days! That means Dynamic Dopamine and Super Serotonin have been releasing happy chemicals in your brain for 20 whole days, *Alhamdulillah!*

What have been your top three Ramadan Alhamdulillah moments these last 20 days? What has made them special?

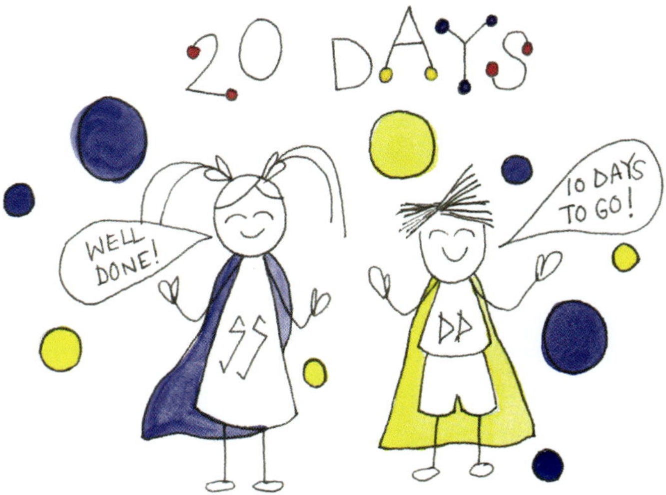
20 DAYS
WELL DONE!
10 DAYS TO GO!
SS
DD

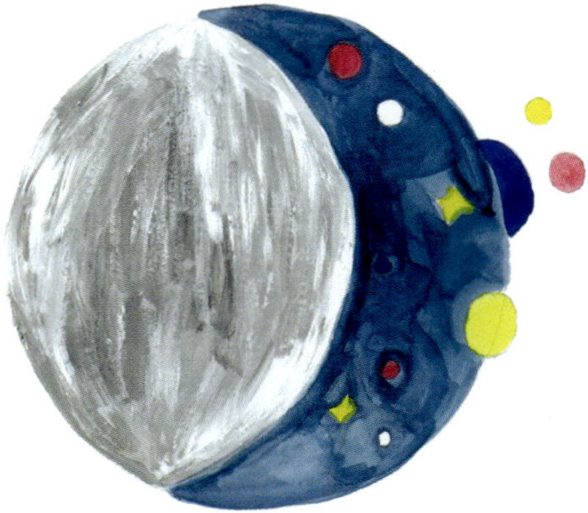

Day 21

Ramadan is a time to pray for our brothers and sisters all over the world. We are all one ummah, which means, Muslim community. Did you know we are a global Muslim community of 1.8 BILLION people? That is phenomenal, *Alhamdulillah!*

Many Muslim children live in unsafe countries. **What message of hope would you like to send them?**

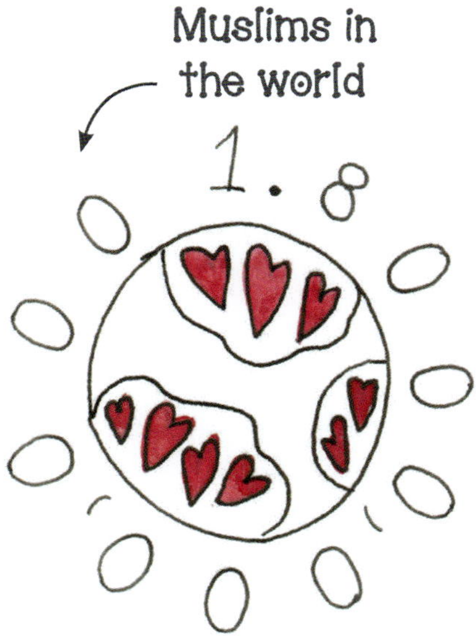

How would you like those in need to **feel** when they read your message? Perhaps you want to tell them that you are praying for them, or that you and your community are going to raise money to help them.

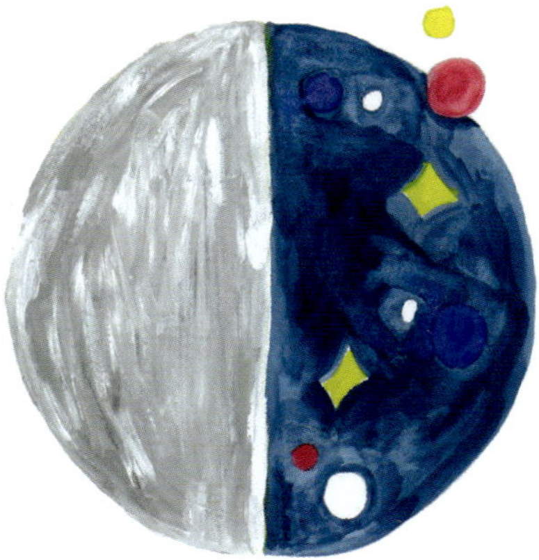

Day 22

Ramadan is a time when we can gain the reward of 70 good deeds just by doing one good deed. *Alhamdulillah* that is super cool!

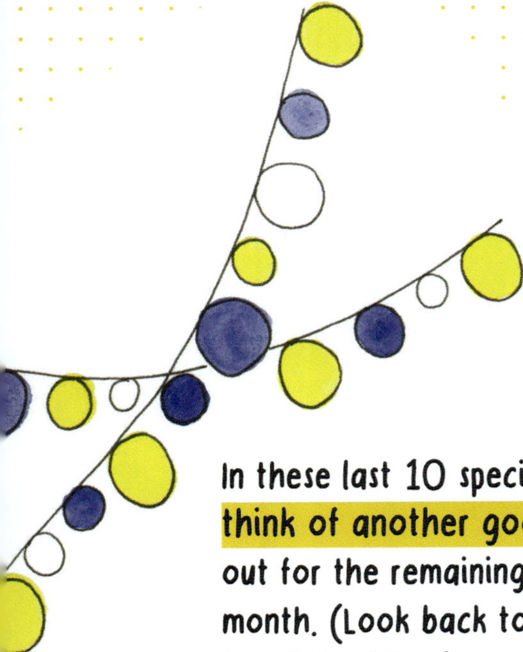

In these last 10 special days of Ramadan, think of another good deed you can carry out for the remaining days of the blessed month. (Look back to our suggestions on Day 3 for ideas).

Make a promise to yourself here:
In these last days of Ramadan, I will try to...

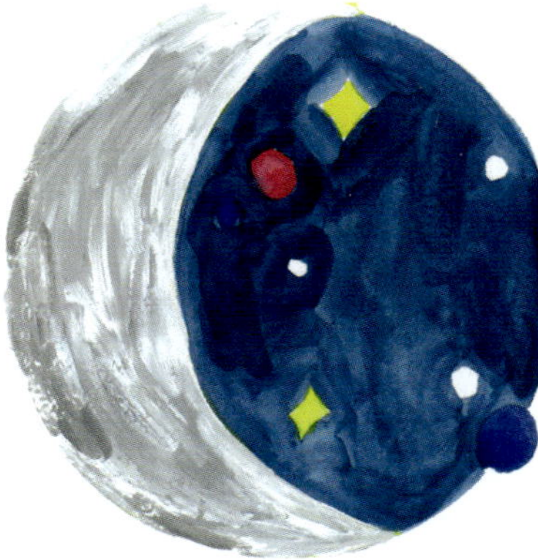

Day 23

Ramadan is a time to show the people who care for us, how much we care for them. We can do this by offering them hugs, which produce more Super Serotonin for them and for us! The more we hug, the happier we feel, *Alhamdulillah!*

Each day, find someone special to hug! You could choose different people for different days.

What would you like them to feel when you hug them? Tell them why you are choosing to hug them and talk about your feelings after you have hugged them.

If they smile because you've hugged them, remember to say, "**Adhakal Lahu Sinnaka**", which means, "May Allah always keep you smiling".

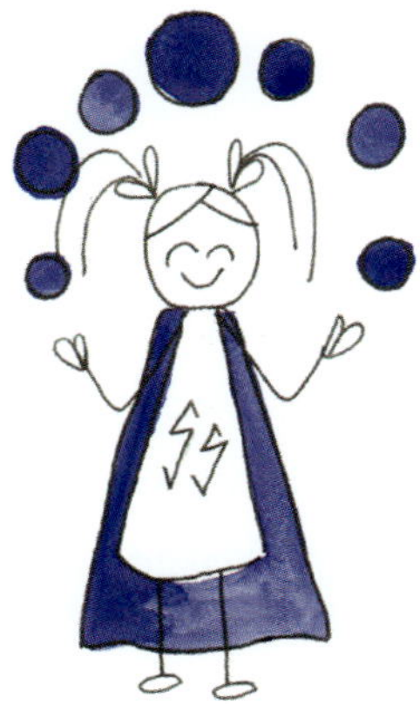

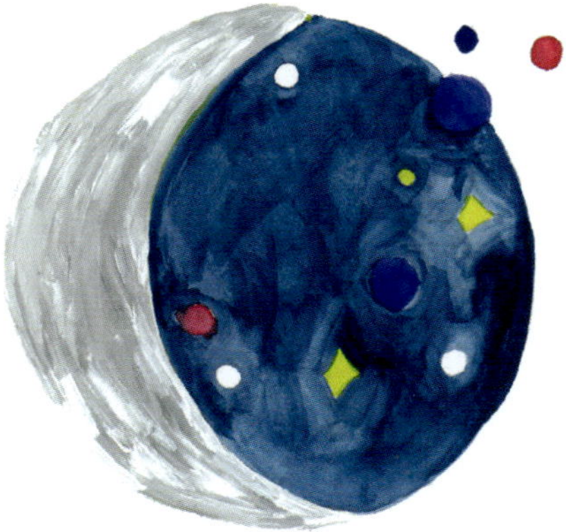

Day 24

Ramadan is a time to read the Qur'an more often, and through this, connect with Allah. The Qur'an is Allah's special book from which we can learn all the miracles that took place in the past, *Alhamdulillah*.

Ask an adult to help you find stories that involve miracles, in the Qur'an. Choose the one that you find most interesting.

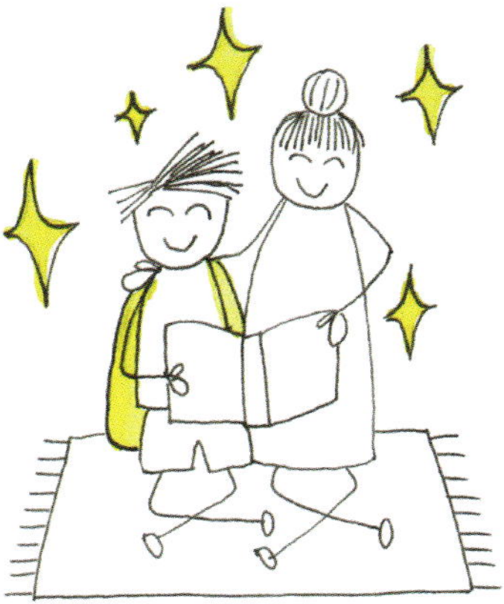

Write down the name of the **surah** and what you found particularly interesting about this miracle.

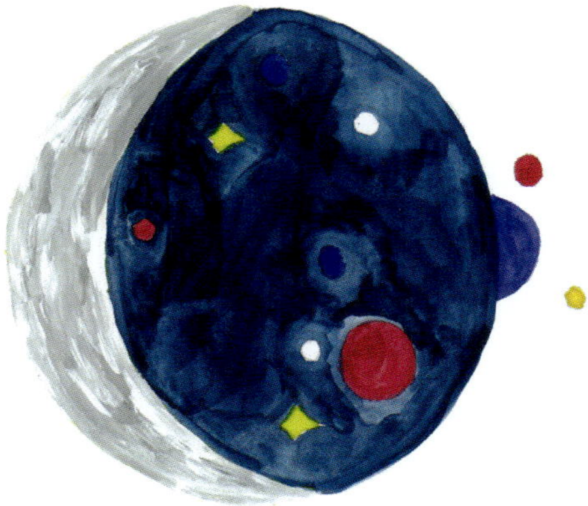

Day 25

Ramadan is a good time to express *shukr* (gratitude) to Allah for all that you have. Finding something to be grateful for, especially when things are tough, will always lift your mood. You can start by being grateful for the ability to be thankful, *Alhamdulillah*.

Think about something in your life that you are grateful for, like a pet, toy, treat or even a person. How does this something or someone special make you feel?

Draw a picture of it here and write a short note to Allah, thanking Him for bringing this personal thing into your life.

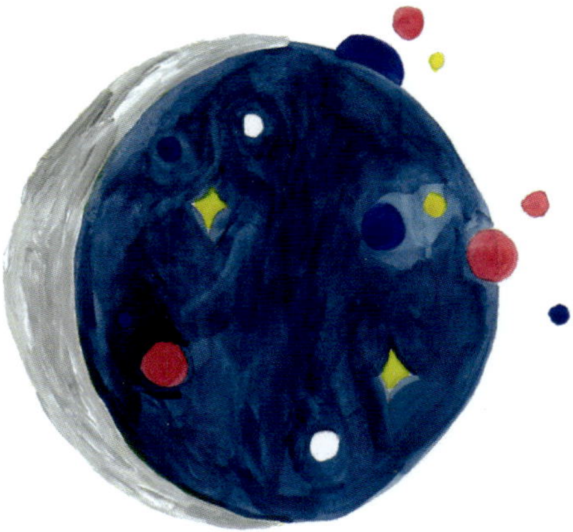

Day 26

Ramadan is a time to try and be better Muslims, both in our actions and in what we say. Saying something nice to encourage someone to feel happy is the easiest way to carry out a good deed. Being kind to others helps us feel happy in ourselves too, *Alhamdulillah*.

Each day, find someone you know to whom you can give a compliment. You can choose a different person for different days.

Choose a compliment by perhaps thinking about things that the person is good at or what you admire or love about them. Remember to say the compliment from your heart.

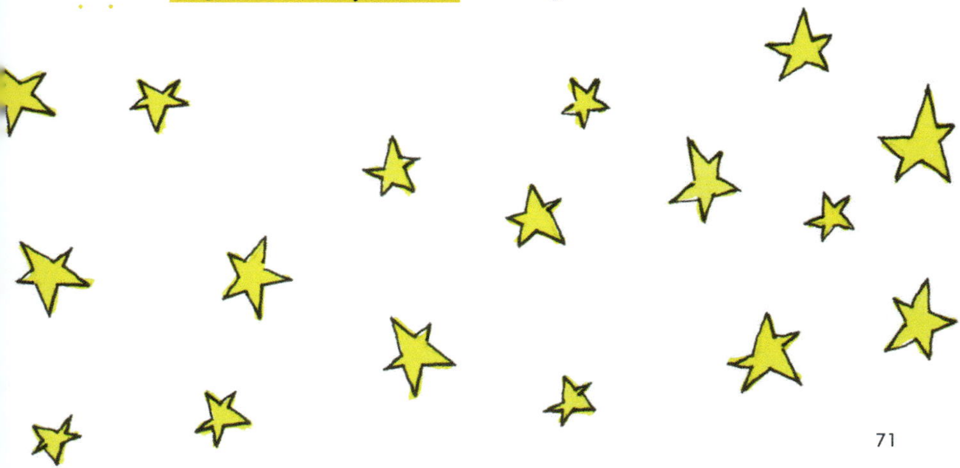

Day 27

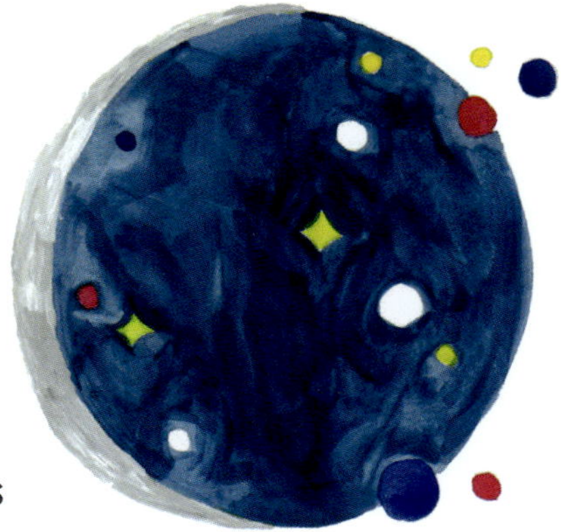

Ramadan is a good time to learn about different Muslim traditions. There are Muslim communities in every country and continent in the World, *MashAllah!* Learning about Ramadan traditions different to our own helps us to have respect and acceptance towards other communities in our big, wide *ummah. Alhamdulillah.*

COOL FACT: Did you also know that appreciating differences in other people, helps you to believe in your own uniqueness too?

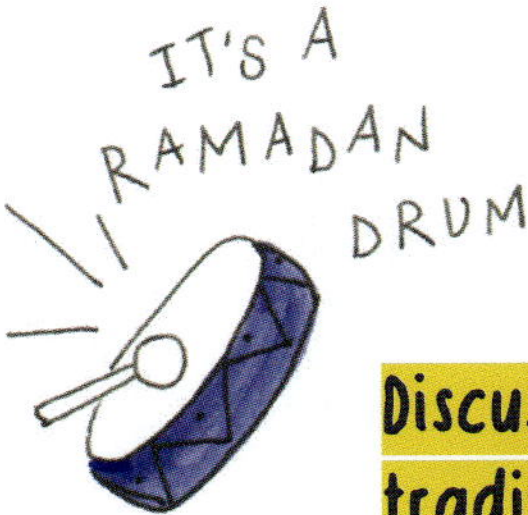

Discuss different Ramadan traditions with a Muslim friend from another culture.

Talk about the traditional foods that are eaten in each community. Are there special clothes that are worn when it's time for prayers?
What things are the same?
What things are different?

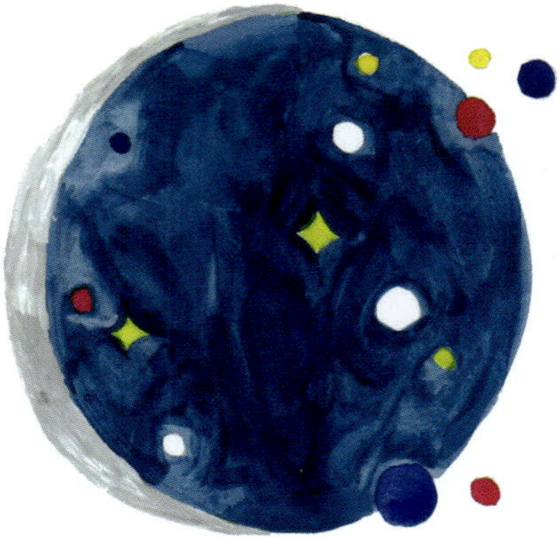

Day 28

Ramadan is a time to thank Allah for all that we have, including how He has made us. Allah made you special and unique! There is only one of you in the world, *Alhamdulillah*.

Can you identify what makes you unique?

Maybe you can roll your tongue... Maybe your pet only comes to you for cuddles... Maybe you can bounce a ball longer than everyone else in your class... Maybe you're amazing at puzzles? Maybe you think about things differently to other people?

Thank Allah for giving you this unique quality to be proud of.

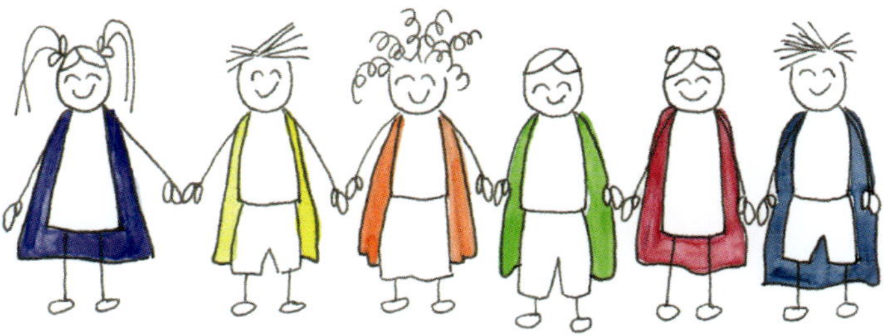

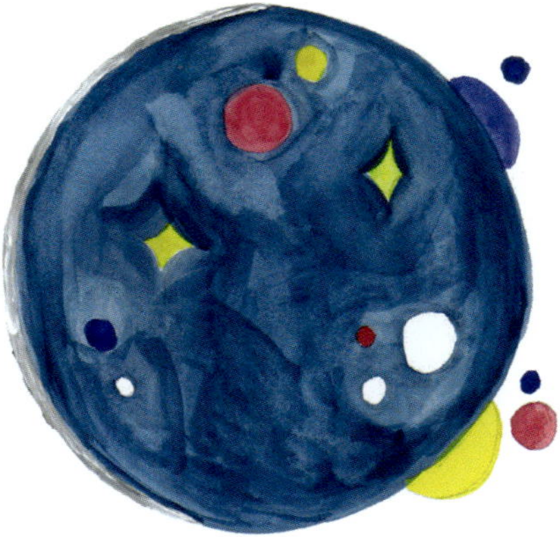

Day 29

Ramadan is a time when we celebrate the festival of Eid. This celebration at the end of the holy month is Allah's way of rewarding us for all our efforts in Ramadan, *Alhamdulillah*.

Think about the people in your home who have worked hard to make sure everyone was looked after in Ramadan.

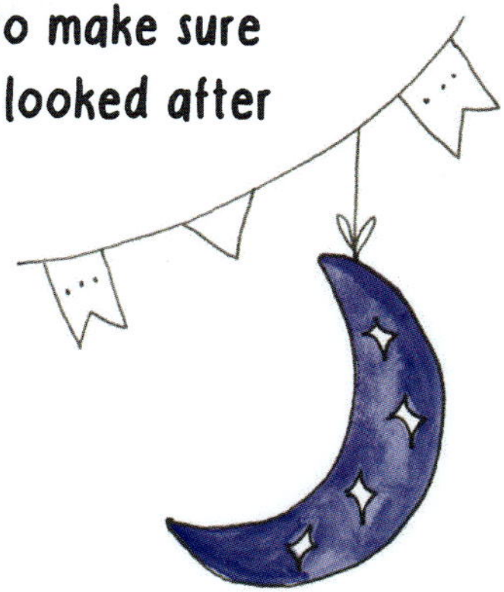

Write them a thank you note or give them a gift to show how much you appreciate their efforts.

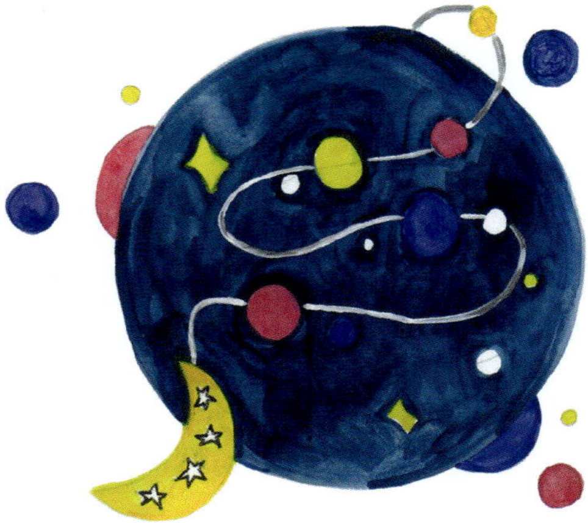

Day 30

Yay! Way to go! You've been practicing gratitude for 30 days! That means Dynamic Dopamine and Super Serotonin have been releasing happy chemicals in your brain for a whole month, *Alhamdulillah!*

Look back at all the wonderful ideas and thoughts you had when reflecting on gratitude this month. Yes! That is what you have been doing for this whole month! Isn't that amazing?

What was your favourite **Alhamdulillah** reflection? Which reflections and practices are you going to carry on with after Ramadan?

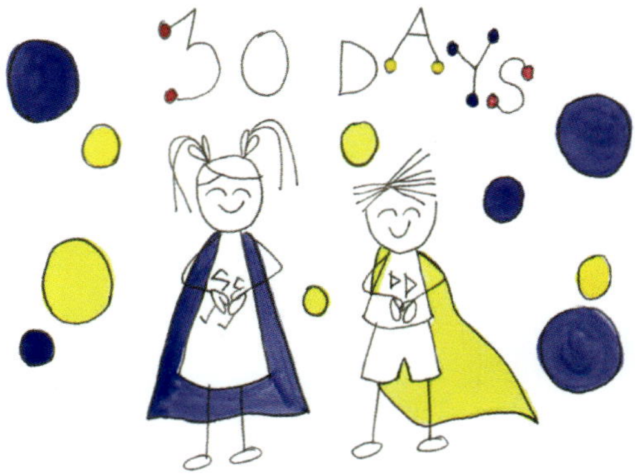

Dynamic Dopamine and Super Serotonin had a great time helping you think about gratitude and special Ramadan *Alhamdulillah* moments. Have you enjoyed it too?

You can come back to this book whenever you like, not just in Ramadan, maybe when you are having a hard time and want to remind yourself about the activities you completed.

Be proud of yourself! Allah is pleased with you for remembering the blessings in your life.

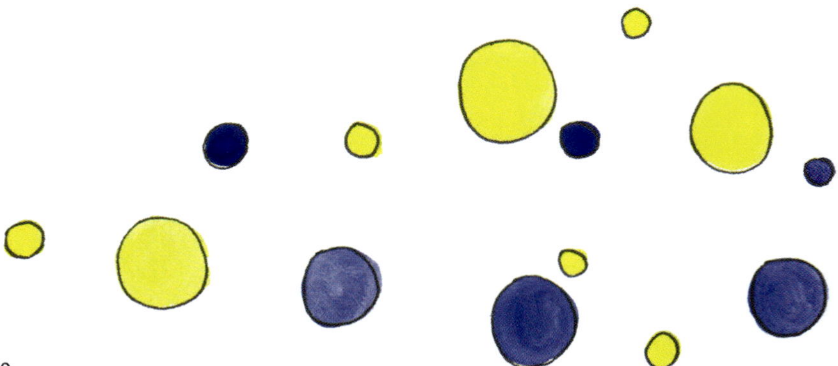

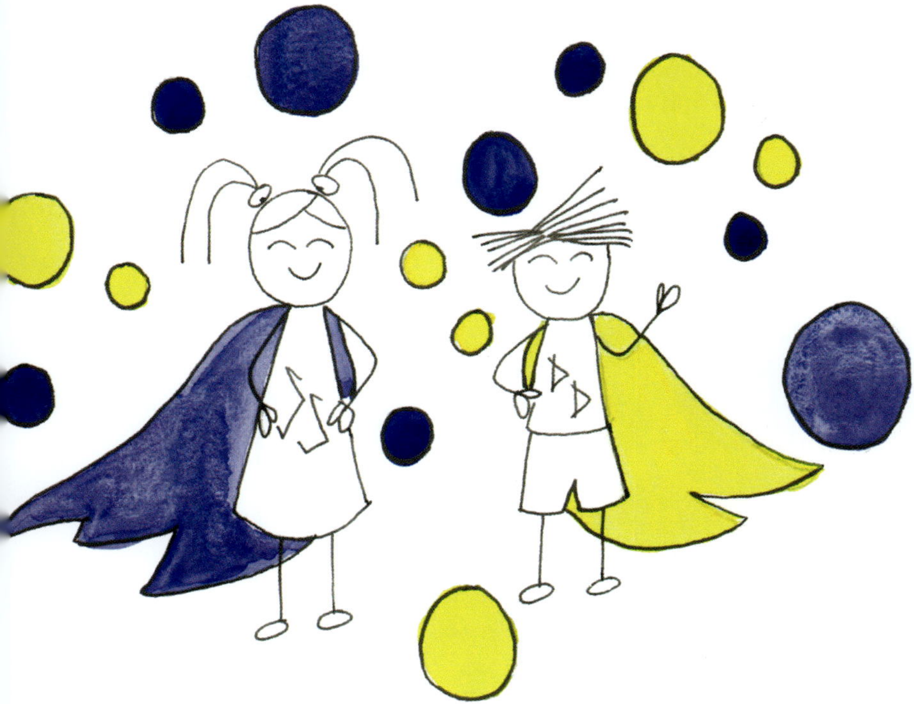

A Note for your Gratitude Buddy

My Ramadan Gratitude moments will help your child:

- Develop a basic understanding of gratitude
- Identify opportunities to cultivate gratitude during the month of Ramadan
- Understand gratitude from a psycho-spiritual perspective by making connections to positive psychology, neuroscience and Islamic principles
- Relate gratitude and its effects on the wider community
- Cultivate God consciousness relating to Allah's attributes as Creator and Giver
- Explore situations and areas of life where gratitude can be practiced as a basis to help formulate their own *Alhamdulillah* moments
- Develop an awareness of difference and acceptance in others
- Encourage self-recognition and improve self-esteem
- Nurture relationships with key figures
- Appreciate that practicing gratitude, even for small things, can help with seeing the world more positively

Our Philosophy

We are a lifestyle brand that is built on the principles of developing emotional, psychological and spiritual wellbeing. Our range of items are expertly curated employing psychology and Islamic faith-based principles. Know that by using our products, you are in good hands.

About the Author

Samia Quddus (MBACP) is a psychotherapeutic Integrative Therapist. She is a specialist practitioner with a background in primary education and Social, Emotional and Mental Health (SEMH). Samia is creator of Taqdeer Life, the UK's first psycho-spiritual Islamic gratitude journal. She is also author of *Freya's Funny Feeling,* a children's story that explores low-level anxiety via the 'butterflies in the tummy' idiom. Her published writing has featured in the British Association for Counsellors and Psychotherapists (BACP) magazine.

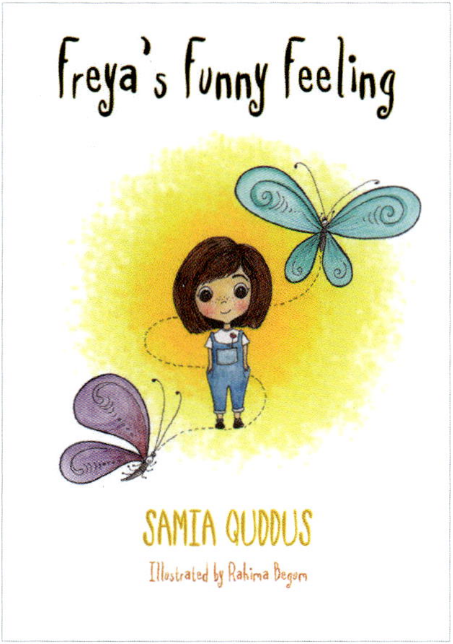

Also by the Author

www.freyasfunnyfeeling.com
hello@freyasfunnyfeeling.com
@freyasfunnyfeeling